BOB MOSS

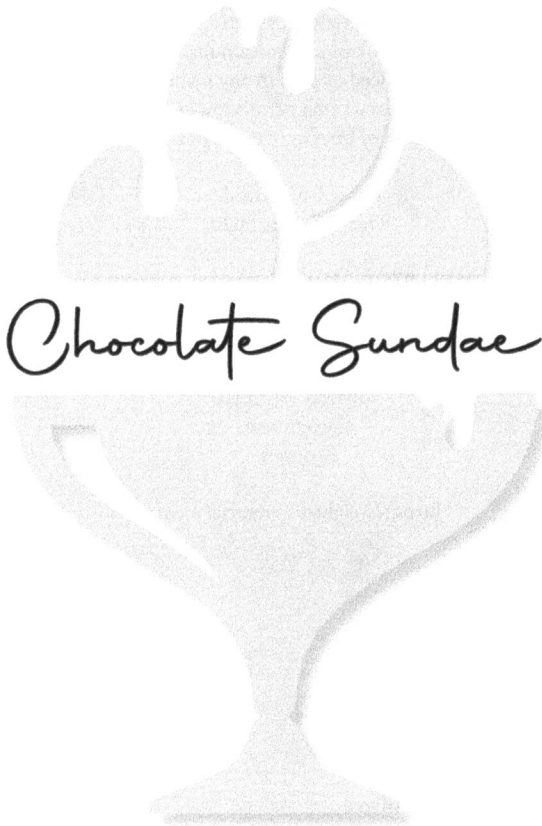

Chocolate Sundae

One man's personal story
of weight loss and reversing diabetes

Printed Worldwide
First Printing, 2020

ISBN 978-0-6450072-0-6 (Paperback)

Bob Moss
PO Box 1747
Runaway Bay 4216
Queensland
Australia

https://weight-loss.management

No Medical or Personal Advice

This book is not intended as a substitute for the medical advice of
physicians. The reader should regularly consult a physician in matters
relating to his/her health and particularly concerning any symptoms that
may require diagnosis or medical attention.

BOB MOSS

Chocolate Sundae

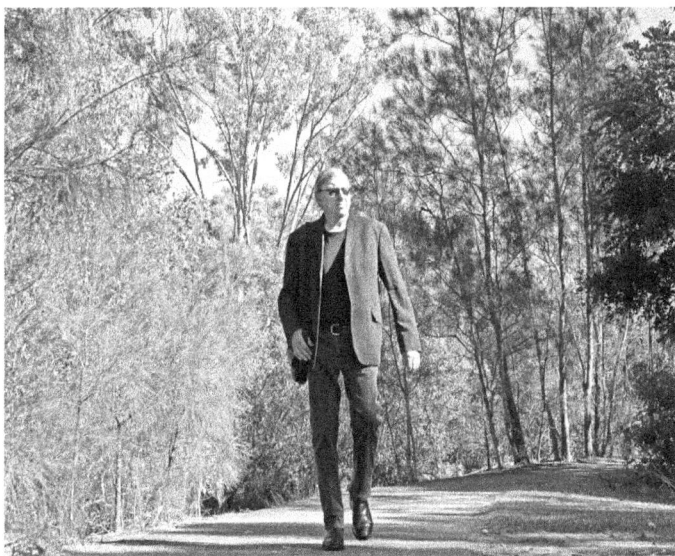

Content

Foreword

I dedicate this book to my whole family, for putting up with my obsessions with most things I do. I'll start with having to get what I want and tending not to see what is going on around me, as I push forward. It includes my trade, at the start of my working life, and the constant need to be the best at what I do. The music where it was not such a success; however, so enjoyable and only killed off by so many band members falling into the pit of never-ending easy drug supply. Then later, my need to read and learn as the obsession of business started to consume me. Add to this my life of travel, and you have a cocktail of a self-centred buggar, who appeared to maybe, not care. All these things add up; built into me is something you cannot see, and that came from my father. That autopilot provided by Frank, my Dad, has been switched on, no matter what, since I was a teen, and that was: *Robert you are here to provide for your family, respect women and "you've made your bed, now lie in it".* All of this forms a big part of my driving force/life. Add to this, the tenacity that came from my Mum.

I do love you all, and this is my official apology. Why? It is because of my shortcomings, so I thank all for your love and patience over all these years. (Oh, and my boating, photographic obsessions, and my new gardening obsession............stop)

Let me finish by saying I am a pure Australian, I love this country with all my soul. There is a spirit here that is indescribable, a look, a smell, a feeling, and it is strong, so I thank the first people for letting us live here. I wish to tell them that we love it and want to protect it just like they do. My Mum Trelly said, there is one word that covers everything in English, "wonderful", Australia is a wonderful place, and all of us that live here are so fortunate.

I would like to make this book short sweet and simple as the saying goes. It may be the smallest book on weight loss and Diabetes ever written. The reason for this book is I want to show that Weight Loss and Diabetes is controllable without really wrecking one's life, and in fact, it may extend one's life.

Chapter One

INTRODUCTION/
WELCOME

Firstly, if you are a Queens English person, put your full harness seatbelt on, as it is going to be a bumpy ride. I would not let the proof-readers take me out of this publication or rearrange the content to make it a best seller. It is what it is, and like modern text messaging, you will adjust to my rhythm as you travel through the chapters. Okay, buckle up!

Let me paint a mental picture: A seventy-year-old man 187.92cm (6' 2") tall, brown hair with some balding happening, fair skin, A friend of his said, *he is looking a bit crusty.* Age is not being kind to this older business guy; the stomach is large like many men at this age, his jeans and suits look untidy due to his weight, his face is full and rounding, again due to weight. He looks tired and a bit sleepy, worn down by years of business travel. If you catch a glimpse of him at the right moment you may see he can't pick things up so well as it is hard to bend over.

And sometimes he has a limp. Some may say, well-worn however; not worn-well. Yes, this was me in 2017.

Why did I write this book? Because something told me I had to help people who were in my situation and did not, or could not, work out the answer. I'm still thrilled about how I did this, even after three years, hence another reason to tell others in my predicament the solution. What happened to me was comparable to a miracle for my health. I just had to let people know. After some advice from a friend, I waited three years to prove this solution worked, as, if I told the story too early, I might not have the proof or trust for the readers. The pandemic provided me with the time to assemble my notes from the three years.

I decided this would not be a technical book with pages of scientific explanations with massive words justifying the writer's authenticity. Also, it would not be a pure diet book ending with imitation recipes of the food that tried to kill me. It had to be my story on how I did what I did, and, if someone can benefit from my experience or emulate it, that will be a good thing.

I looked at book after book and there where chapter after chapter giving the medical reasons for weight gain and Diabetes: the different types of sugar there are, graphs and many medical terms. Just dull stuff where you get tired reading it, as there is nothing you can do with this knowledge, that is if you could understand it. I don't care about fructose and can never remember its role in all the weight analysis jargon.

I planned to assemble the book so the reader could see my life and how I got myself into and out-of-the situation that many others may have found themselves in. When the reader arrives at the end of the book, they will fully understand how I went about this. In the last pages of the book, like a manual, I have put the steps to my success in bullet points, so there is no flicking back to see what I did at certain stages of my journey.

You can see a bit of business experience comes into this, with focus, planning and outcomes. (More about my business life later in the book).

I believed I had an audience in my head for the book, and I think, it may not be correct as there are many in my western society, I know, who need someone's story so they can act themselves and do something about the situation they have found themselves in. I am a baby boomer, and there are plenty of respondents in this category who will have been travelling the same road I have been on, consequently this group, may benefit from this read. This following dialogue will prove, that, no matter the age, young to old, it is never too late to act.

Some will say I am not qualified to write on this subject, I say, you reckon! My retort is, okay have you detractors reversed Diabetes, lost weight, had health checks and blood tests that are all normal, plus sustained this success for over three years? Oh, you have not? I rest my case, sir/madam.

The whole thing is simple when you break it down, my food intake is now simple, my exercise is simple, my stress is minimal, and my enjoyment has been immense since I made the changes I did, read on........

Chapter Two

MY UPBRINGING STORY
(BACKGROUND)

Please don't think I was an angel, I was a bad boy, a wild boy, fast cars, wild music and bands, surfing risk taker, women problems, police concerns and I was single minded and stubborn to top it off. Yet I made it through my teens alive, how I don't know?

This first section of the book in a way proves, what you put in with your kids eventually, comes out the other end.

In my case, much, much later. That is, what you feed the family, how you educate them, the example you set daily and how and where to get a discount, maybe. I am a result of my upbringing—some outcomes examples, education, manners, diet and honesty, to name a few. Most everything about me came from my home and school. We may group this into values if you like. All of this brings me to the main point, of all the things in my life; I am most grateful for is the gift my parents gave me, my upbringing.

I'm a Catholic boy raised in Lane Cove, Sydney Australia. I came from a family of six children. My Mother was an excellent cook and had to be, due to the family's size. When you have a family this size, food is a big deal, normal meals, gatherings for Christmas birthdays anniversaries and so on. Food in our size family was never-ending and had to have production and clean-up methods. It did have methods, and it worked and did so for years with a kind of unwritten roster.

Probably some downfalls in later life were from being brought up on an English diet. This English diet included sweets/desserts after every main meal. I'm not blaming here, as it was merely traditional and of course, the whole family loved a desert. It was good tucker, three veg, meat and potatoes and then something like a lemon meringue pie to finish off the meal. Yum! Being Catholic, it was Fish and Chips from the Lane Cove Fish and Chip Shop on a Friday. (As short return bike trip from home)

We were all very healthy, at that time before iPads and iPhones. Exercising was not a concern as we were all vibrant kids; no parents were driving us to schools during those days. Times were good, and freedom for kids was not an issue……….. just disappear and come home at mealtimes. Our home area in Lane Cove at that time, was bush or forest/wood for those worldwide readers. As young boys we had treehouses, rock fights, Cicada catching, blackberry picking, tadpole catching, swimming in the Harbour, bicycle riding, billy cart racing, pet Blue Tongue Lizards and the list goes on, sounds good? *It* was! Strangely we rarely saw any killer Brown Snakes or Funnel-Web Spiders although it was notorious for these in that part of Sydney. We were fortunate to avoid these two hazards as we spent many hours in the bush around where we lived. (Did I mention the Bushfires, they sometimes came close)

I was very mechanically minded, and my destiny was going to be in the motor industry as the first word I said to my Mother was, "Car". My academic skills were limited, and it was only in midlife, I discovered, that I was dyslexic, my only other minor issue, was that I was red green colour-blind like my father, this meant no pilot licence ever.

I disliked school mainly because the teachers didn't like me as I appeared to be dumb to them. When you have trouble with spelling and maths, it frustrates the teachers, and they lose patience with you. I was never really educated until I did it myself, as no one at that time could teach a person with dyslexia, so we were scrap heaped, "yep, dunces". My first school was a drama as the Nuns disliked me as they saw me as stupid/dumb. My first school day I wet my pants in the playground as I just did not fit, it was a lonely place for me. Later a Nun took a real dislike to me and would lock me in the classroom at mealtimes, I'll say it, "what a bitch!!!!". Many nights I would secretly cry myself to sleep, lonely again because of lack of fitting in. My Mum changed my school and the American Nuns were much kinder to me. This was a huge change. The hate for school came back in the higher grades, high school, as the teachers turned on me again. I somehow adjusted, to the continued abuse over my inability to learn and by some means it gave me a weird strength that help me cope, even though to them, I was, the fool on the hill (Lennon–McCartney). Humour became my internal weapon, I could see the funny side of people opposite me, the stupid habits they had, their looks, hair and dress, speech, or walk. In other words, how can you judge me when you are so stupid yourself? Handy tool later in corporate situations I have to say, as no one can see what you are really thinking in some really stupid business situations. This gift taught me to look into people and situations, a very good tool to possess.

Today I still have no concerns with solitude as I did in

my younger days. I learnt it was okay, as it kept me away from the school bully's. In fact, solitude taught me the advantages of time for deep thinking. I guess that is why I have been able to travel easily worldwide, by myself, for extensive business trips, alone in hotel rooms is normal and easy for me. I am very productive alone once the house is quite and everyone has bedded down for the night.

Being dyslexic you find creative ways to get around everything, and this helps your mind. You also need a good memory so that you can get out of embarrassing situations. In simple terms, your creativity has to compensate, so it grows. My mechanical ability was excellent. I can dismantle and reassemble an alarm clock without any problems. I was obsessed with cars and had many toy model cars. (I still stop in the toy departments and look at diecast model cars) Cars fascinated me, and my Dad was always working on his cars doing repairs such as head gaskets, valve grinds, oil changes, tyre changes, fitting accessories like Towbars, so I was a continuous observer. Hence, being car crazy, I became a Motor Mechanic and a good one. (Technician). These mechanical skills put all that drama at school behind me, and I was super happy not to look in the rear vision mirror. Some other skills I discovered were; that I could drive well, swim well and could sing in tune. With these skills, I did well, I could make money at work and fixing cars at home. Besides I could sing, girls liked that, and I liked girls. Money, Cars, Surfboards, Music the teenage years were excellent, and I am smiling when I think back to those days. My positivity arrived and has never departed.

I did not know I was dyslexic until my mid-forties. I believe I was lucky to be oblivious to my condition as I had noth- ing to wallow in so I was just determined to prove to the detractors, that I could do anything they said I could not. Stuff them!!!!! The secret to success is doing what you love, in my case again, Cars, Business, the Water, Music, Computers, Gardening..............and the meas- urement for success is simply you enjoy it!

Finally, on this theme, why is being a dyslexic relative to my diet? Because I taught myself to break everything down to its simplest form, so I could understand it, be it automotive electronics that I taught at one time or a Low-Carb diet. So, I hope in this book I have peeled everything back so all can see the simplicity and the practicality of what I discovered. I am also driven by anyone saying I will not succeed; I almost love it. In 2003 a gentleman said I would never succeed as a consultant. It has driven me ever since!!! This dates to the teachers telling me the same, *you are going* nowhere. Just a hint of someone telling me that Low-Carb would not work and away I went. Bring it on I say!!

My Dad finished up an accountant in the Government, and he would teach us business stuff of a night. It was so dull/boring; however, some of my Dad's skills rubbed off as I have worked with automotive financials for many years and still do so today. See, what you put into your kids comes out later. My best subject at school was Business Principles. Back then it never crossed my mind it was a skill, I thought it was a mistake that I passed in this subject, I find it amusing now as it finished up being my life.

Chapter Three

IF THEY COULD SEE ME NOW

(MATURING)

I was married at 22 and had two girls before I was 30, moved to Adelaide and worked three jobs to buy a house. It was a hard life, yet, I made it through and was promoted and finished up working for Ford Motor Company head office in Adelaide. I worked my way up through the industry educating myself along the way as I was the only one who could teach me. It's still the same today, I still love learning. I grin when I think of those teachers who gave me "shit" and had no time to help a wretch like me. (Some of those teachers were "bastards" believe me, in some cases downright cruel) I eventually became a Senior Executive in the car industry. This work took me around and around the world. (What is that song: Sweet Charity - 'If They Could See Me Now')

Over this long period and after giving up smoking in

my early thirties, I was continually fighting off weight and blood pressure problems. I did this through dieting and exercise, and it's safe to say that I have exercised most of my life. I got to a point where the Doctor told me to start walking and stop running as I was wearing out my joints. The exercise certainly worked reducing my blood pressure. Every time I stopped exercising, the blood pressure (BP) went back up, when I was exercising the BP dropped back to normal without medication. There is a lesson in the previous sentence on blood pressure, best make a note on this.

You can imagine that once you reach Executive level things become different, life is all about food, out to dinner, out to lunch and eating junk food on aeroplanes and in airports. It's a foodathon: everything seems to revolve around food. Also, there is as much alcohol as you want to drink, and it is the best quality available. Fortunately, I do not drink much at all; otherwise, it would have been crazier than what it was in terms of weight control.

All this time I knew that I had to do something, however trying to find out what to do, and when, was difficult, that may be an excuse. I guess in some ways it was like smoking, trying to give up is a massive task as many of you know. The temptation to smoke again was always there, as when I did smoke that kept the weight down, and I used it for relaxing when things in life got tough.

No matter what path you travel in Western Society that trail ends up at food, bring a plate, go to a school fate, visit friends, BBQ's, morning teas for the staff, school function, corporate body breakfasts, think about it, you can't escape. Here have a little more, it's delicious, come on, there is plenty left over get stuck in, take some home with you for a snack later. Sugar everywhere, intertwined into the food somehow, be it, the elderly lady down the road giving away her cakes or a sneaky food producer covering it up with the word Lite (Light) on the packet.

So that is my life up until a short time ago when the diagnosis came in that I had Type Two Diabetes.

Before we move on, you should know the story about how I learnt about focus and how to set goals then achieve them, plus the feeling of achieving those goals; this plays a large part in my success with losing weight and reversing Diabetes.

Chapter Four

FOCUS/GOALS/
ACHIEVEMENT/MONEY
AND A CHOCOLATE
SUNDAE

When I was about ten years old, I started to discover the value of money and the feeling of freedom. I went to Lane Cove Primary School in Sydney. For those who are interested, Nicole Kidman went there many years after me. I suppose she did not know or care about that tall, skinny kid who sat at that desk before her, learning nothing and thinking about cars (Matchbox toys at that time).

Yes, I am still thinking about cars; some things don't change. As I stated earlier, I was such a disappointment to my Mum. Most little boys' first word is "Ma Ma". My first word was "car". That day when I told Mum what I was thinking, absolutely set the direction for my life. Poor Mum; what did she think on that day, and I was not an easy baby, as I understand it. Mum is in heaven now probably telling that story to another angel (bless her).

My first recollection of the pleasure that money can bring came not long after my first job. I discovered I needed cash if I wanted more diecast matchbox toys, and a new bike. There were only two ways to make money, work for money or steal it. (Catholic boys don't steal stuff) Don't get me wrong, as I am not promoting money as a God here. Just be honest with yourselves as you read this, as we all know the pleasure when we buy things. (Don't we!) In sales, they call it "wants and needs" self-explanatory don't you think. You know the wants are the ones I am talking about here. A footnote on this paragraph, I am no longer a Catholic boy; only on paper, some disconcerting life experiences cured me of religion, don't worry, no one ever touched me up, and I still stick by the rules that were drilled into me as a little kid, "don't steal anything Robert".

Fortunately, or maybe not, I won a job doing what they called a Chemist Run (drugstore in the USA). Someone in the family had heard about the position or seen a notice in the Chemist Shop window. I went to see the Head Chemist one afternoon when school finished. It was a gruelling interview. I asked, "do you have a job for a Chemist Delivery Boy?", and the guy said, "yep, when do you want to start?" He went on, "I'll try you out for a week if you can do it you can stay. If not, its hasta la vista". He was ahead of his time as the movie came years later. He continued, "Its two bucks a week that includes Saturday mornings". I started that day. I lasted the first week, so I turn into a permanent Super Chemist Delivery Boy, and I'll tell you it felt good.

My new job was to deliver prescription drugs to the retired people in Lane Cove. Retired people made up about half the population of Lane Cove at that time, and it is still the same today I would think; a mini Florida. It was like slave labour. If you know Lane Cove, it is all hills, and some bloody big ones near Sydney Harbour. Rain, hail, storms or cold, for two hours after school, in my grey school shorts on my bike I would deliver these lifesaving drugs to the elderly of Lane Cove.

It was not unlike that saying, "The Mail Must Go Through". I do not know how many lives I saved for that miserable $2.00 per week; however, it would be over one hundred, I reckon. Did anyone care? I don't think so. The wage calculation was 0.4cents a minute. Thinking back maybe I was not that smart; however, I did get smarter later, thankfully.

I would go in at 3:15 pm, and they would give me my

first deliveries. Away I would go zooming through the traffic at top speed, dodging Holden (GM) taxis that came from the Taxi rank near the chemist shop. I had my leather carry bag on the rear bike-rack, which securely protected the valuable cargo of lifesaving drugs for the retirees. My blue semi racing bike with the chrome wheels flashing in the afternoon sunlight and the reflections of that beautiful blue Sydney Harbour at Longueville, dancing off the shiny rims. No 'Occupation Health and Safety rules' in this game. It was every boy for himself. After riding across Lane Cove to Longueville and back, they would give me my next Job – 'What the Fuck', a delivery almost next door to where I had just been. There was no system or process in this place. Off I would go again, and every so often I would get a tip of 50cents. Those oldies in Lane Cove were not good at parting with their money. The Chemist Boss said we had to declare the tip's, no way.......... 'Fuck' him! Boys with bikes were plentiful. Kill one-off in the traffic, and there were another ten to take his place for two bucks a week, including Saturday's. Much like when I was in Corporate....... kill one-off with stress, and there was another to take his/her place.

Now, there had to be some pleasure after all this work, and I found it. Another Chemist boy explained to me what a Chocolate Sundae was and where to get them, I was so interested as it almost sounded illegal. He presented it like it was drugs. The place to buy these was the tuck shop/milk-bar right next to Lane Cove Primary School. (Nicole would know it) So I went to school early on a Monday morning after my first Chemist Run payday on Saturday.

With the money in my pocket I nervously went to the counter and asked for a Chocolate Sundae. I then sat in the cubicle, and they brought the Sundae over to me, Wow! I can still taste it today as I write this. There were three Scoops of pure white Ice-Cream stacked in the centre of the wine glass shaped dish; the Ice-Cream formed a white mountain, The beautiful dark chocolate cascading like a volcano erupting over the top of the ice-cream and down the sides. There were nuts sprinkled on the top of the chocolate. A small spoon protruded from the side of the Ice-Cream, it looked too perfect for eating, almost. It sure sounds illegal as I write this, so much pleasure and no punishment. I don't think there has ever been anything that tasted so good ever since that day. It was a combination of things: the freedom of being able to go in there with my own money and have the Sundae: it was brought to me at the cubicle in the Tuck Shop/Milk Bar: and I was now living the life. (I wonder if Nicole experienced that same pleasure. I guess she did.) And yes, it was sugar, that was the poison that would try to kill me later in life. It's sad. so sad, it's a sad sad situation! (*Elton John*) Don't worry I'm not off message, I am just leading into the sugar/diabetes/weight subject, as some parts of my life are relevant, as to how I got myself into, then out of, this horrid health situation.

My next step into this murky world of pleasure was cigarettes……….. let's not go there!

Not far from the chemist shop, there was a type of electrical shop. They sold radios and all kinds of strange stuff. The guys in this shop would do things like listening to short-wave radio, (amateur radio operators) picking up BBC and telling everyone the next day what they heard, for example: the Queen's Christmas message, and things like that, I guess. (No, I was after Winston Churchill). The electrical shop catered for these amateur radio operators with the items they needed for their hobbies. We see those big satellite TV dishes on house roofs today; it is a similar hobby I believe; they were tuning into overseas television broadcasts.

One day when passing this shop, on the way to save the elderly of Lane Cove again, I spotted what looked like a small radio. On looking closer, it was a "crystal set" which is a thing that somehow picks up radio waves; it did not need batteries and came with a single earphone. This one looked a lot like a pocket radio; it was very modern for that time. I was in love with it at first sight, much like today when I see new Apple or Surface laptop computers. (You can buy the Crystal Radio Kits on eBay or other sites today if you are interested.) Now my focus was set. It would take me about five weeks of lifesaving work to buy that radio, so that was my goal. (A want......... not a need) I worked and waited, checking every day to see if it was still there, much like watching eBay today. I went without "chocolate sundaes" in this period, that was not easy. Then the big day came, and it was still there. I went into the store and asked the old guy if I could buy the radio. He went to the shop window and retrieved it from its prominent place in the display, putting it in the original box. I handed over the money and received the Crystal Set.

I rode the blue bike home, very fast, as I had to try out the new and first serious item I had ever purchased. Can you imagine the excitement? It was a wonder I did not crash going down what we called the Big Black Hill. I sat on the bottom bunk in our bedroom and started turning the dial and tuning in to the stations. The sound travelled down that skinny braided wire to the earplug. It worked............ and as night came, it worked even better. It was an early Walkman and excellent. (I must admit it, about 6 years ago I purchased a crystal set, the same model, from eBay. It now sits on the shelf in my office to remind me of my background and helps me on 'how to focus.'

I had many hours of pleasure from that little Crystal Set (the forerunner to the iPod, I guess). The reason we had a bunk bed was there were three of us (brothers) in the one room. At that time, I had the bottom bunk. (Col and I still play music together.) What a fantastic brother he is. Sadly, Bruce, my other brother passed away at a young age of 28 [Bruce played bass]. Bruce is still there some nights when the music is rocking.

I learned much from that small part of my life:

- It's alright to have a vision and a goal, and if you believe it, it can come true, I dreamed of listening to that radio.
- You can have what you want, but you must work hard for it. You have to plan, focus and set goals, or you will not get what you want or need. (*Rolling Stones, You Can't Always Get What You Want*)
- You have to go without sometimes to get what you want.
- The feeling of achievement is a better feeling than

the taste of a chocolate sundae.
- The value of money and that you must work hard for it.
- How fast the money goes/disappears.
- You can gain pleasure from material things and if you worked hard for it, why not?
- I learnt I had a value, and it was $2.00 per week.

This value was because:

> I could communicate well.
> I could count so I could collect money.
> I was healthy.
> I could ride a bike.
> I had an excellent work ethic.
> I was reliable.

Later I learnt:

- I was a poor negotiator, as I took the first wage offered to me by the Chemist.
- I learnt about how business works and how the money goes around.
- I also learnt that the Chemist was ripping me off and that selling newspaper was a much better job with improved pay.

I moved to a job selling newspapers outside the Lane Cove Pub on Saturday evenings. I made five times the wage on one night per week as the patrons were drunk, and the tips were excellent. I could get a base wage of $5.00 for Saturday evening (about 3 hours of work) plus tips.

Here is what I learnt from this:

- To shop the market for jobs and not take the first offered.
- Because I had a job, I could get another one.
- The experience was valuable.
- My track record with collecting money with the Chemist shop was second to none.
- I could present my skills and attributes.
- I learnt that my value in the marketplace could go up as I had the experience.
- The more money I could make the boss, the more he would pay me, and the more someone else would want me to work for them.
- I learnt to take a risk.

The above gave the Paper Shop confidence to employ me. The time spent as a child slave at the chemist shop did have some value. It got me the experience and education I needed to improve. Then my personal value had increased. I had never sold a newspaper in my life before, so I tried and succeeded.

The story is to show that all those basic things we learn about business are correct - planning, goal setting and achievement. As a Manager, I emulated those feelings of accomplishment many times, and now as a business owner, I still do it the same way as the kid in the grey shorts on the bike, or outside the pub. It is no different; it all still works the same way. I just don't save as many lives these days as I did then, although I have helped save a few businesses.

The overall point is that if you educate yourself, no matter what age you are, you can increase your value to someone else. All the things I learned way back then, still apply today. Work hard and learn to think and take a risk. Educate yourself; no one else will help you. Being too comfortable kills your learning and your spirit. I have seen too many friends give up and stop learning and that to me is the start of dying. A loss of interest is the worst disease you can get.

I did all this, yet, like many things in life, I did not realise I was doing a lot of it naturally; probably because my Dad was business-minded. Once I could understand it, I could focus more on refining such things as focus, goals, education in my specialised areas etc.

For those who don't know Lane Cove, it is now one of the better suburbs in Sydney. It was not so classy back then. It is just north of the Harbour and is beautiful with lots of trees and greenery. We were very fortunate to have grown up in that peaceful, safe place where Mum did not have to worry about us. We would go down to the bush to play in the morning, come back for lunch and home for dinner. We all wish that life today was this simple, alas there are too many weirdo's around stuffing it up for all of us.

In this section of the book, I have explained some of my business life as it gave me the ability and base to focus and fight my new life battle, with health. It has allowed me to live a little longer here on planet earth. I hope what I have written assists you to gear up and focus on your health battles.

Chapter Five

WEIGHT LOSS AND DIABETES
(GETTING TO THE NITTY-GRITTY)

So here we go, on weight loss and Diabetes. My strong business background gave me many of the appropriate tools in setting goals and achieving what I had to so I could live longer. You may be able to emulate this. The other part of this story is understanding where and how I got myself to where I was and how to reverse it if I could. And finally, the essential part that strangely is also something that we have to use in business, and that is 'sustainability'. No more of this weight on, weight off, 'Yo-yo'. Sustainability has been proven for and by me; hence I can now write about it with confidence, so many weight loss successes appear and then disappear without a word NOT THIS ONE!!!!

As you will appreciate, I write this from a male perspective (I am a male so I must), however, ladies, please make the necessary female interpretations for me and transpose the viewpoints where appropriate. Next, tell your partners what you have learned from these writings.

I am well-adjusted and I'm happily married, and I am a powerful advocate for women and more of them in my male-dominated Motor Vehicle industry, now we have the record straight.

Here are my notes before commencing my journey in May 2017. It is what I felt and thought before learning how to do something about correcting my health and life.

- I hated the way I looked in the mirror, especially my stomach.

- I could rest stuff on my stomach like I was pregnant. My stomach was like a little TV dinner table.

- Nothing fitted me anymore, my suit and sports jackets did not do up because my stomach was too big, so I was buying bigger clothes to cover up my fat.

- My belts were all too small.

- I could not see my appendage anymore. (Sorry, yet it's true!

- My snoring was shocking.

- I had trouble putting my shoes on and cutting my toenails.

- When I bent over it made me short of breath.

- I would become out of breath, climbing stairs and walking up hills.

- I exercised. Nothing happened to my weight. It stayed the same or dropped slightly…….. then came back up or increased.

- I was always hungry 1 hour after a meal and wanted more food, snacks, sugary stuff.

- Sometimes I'd feel weak, so I'd suck some Barley-Sugar to reduce the fatigue.

- I purchased 'lite' everything, and it did not help at all.

- I was tired all the time, sleepy.

- I was swelling up more and more, especially my legs.

- When I walked, I suffered chafing at the top of my legs.

- My blood pressure was always high, so I needed more medication; it was difficult to control.

- I experienced acid stomach badly at times, and I still

do suffer from this; however, my large stomach helped the acid increase in the esophagus. I'd wake in the night from acid burning my throat.

- I was feeling like a loser, as, no matter what I did; it would not work. This knowledge came with some depression.

- Inside I knew the weight was killing me; still, all roads led to nowhere. Strangely in some type of 'protest', I would give up and eat more, especially sugar-based food.

- I read labels in the supermarket and would try to eat products with less sugar. It did not work, and I could not work out why.

- I was sneaky and would buy a packet or two of peanuts M&M's when I purchased fuel for the car in the service (gas) station.

- I would look at others who looked like me, and I wished that I did not look like that side on.

- My head was never clear, and my concentration was less than ever before.

- I now had Diabetes (maybe borderline), and I was pricking my fingers doing blood tests four times a day.

The stuff I was eating and taking was not working. In other words, the blood sugar levels were still high and spiked very high at times.

- The diabetes medication made me dizzy, and I would feel nauseous from it.

- I disliked having my photo taken as I hated how I looked.

- People kept telling me that as you get older, you can't lose weight as the young ones can.

My willpower was exhausted so that I would go back to my old ways after each diet, and I become heavier. It was like I had a death-wish………….yet I did not!

As you can see, I was a mess. I never let it show in the business world. I am usually a very positive person. However, this was pushing me to the limit. I was walking 5km a day. I did this for six months before I started my new journey. This 5km a day programme I had set myself did zip, nothing!!! My 115kg just sat there, and my blood pressure did not reduce, as it had always done before when I did regular exercise. I was fucked, using one of my old motor-mechanic terms. I had reached a stage where I could not see a way out of this, and it looked like I was heading to be a huge unhealthy guy, a bit sad, don't you think?

Back then, I had been advised I was heading to becoming a diabetic, and my life would be cut short. Yes, that was me. All the items in the list above were me that is how I know how to write this so; clearly. I've been there, I was there, and I am no longer there. HARRAH!

The main thing here as a reader is who do you believe when it comes to losing weight, and you have a lifetime sentenced as a person with Diabetes, so you are stuck with that. So, can you trust me, yes, why, I have been where you are at now, and I am now Diabetes free, besides my stomach has gone just some excess flab leftover now?

Therefore, here is my first rule; there was no exercise in the first three months, it was too hard for me to drag that body around, it was better to lose the weight first and then start my exercise. Now that's a rule you did not expect.

You see those TV programs where some people are almost killing themselves doing idiotic things with some guy or girl shouting at them. If that happened to me, I would walk away as I can't stand people dominating with those types of bully/army methods. If I did not walk away, I would probably have a heart attack from the extremes they go to, to get the kilograms off. Guess what, as soon as I stopped any of my exercise programs, my weight returned, and my list of items that I hated about myself also returned, step by step and it happened quickly. As I become older, I just can't do that heavy exercise stuff anymore; however, I keep moving walking, gardening, fixing things and boating.

Chapter Six

SENTENCING TO THEN FREEDOM

Weight and Diabetes run hand in hand so I need to tell you this part of my story as some may be going where I have gone before, (*sounds like StarTrack going where no man has gone before*), this chapter may put the brakes on someone else's journey, I hope this is a short cut or a gift, I can give away. If you are a Type Two Diabetic, one hundred percent, read on.

I was a borderline Type Two Diabetic for years. I believed the answer was to stop sugar, so I did, and the weight fell off, even though I kept off the sugar the weight gradually came back over about a year. I added more exercise, that didn't work, no loss of weight happening at all. Why? I'm doing everything correctly was running around in my head, it was so frustrating? I could not work it out everything in the fridge and pantry was lite/low fat, I checked every label for Sugar/Fat/Trans-Fat and always took the lowest sugar content products. I was very irritated as the sugar was gone and the reverse was happening................... the weight was coming back?

To continue the story of discovery regarding my health. I was travelling at the time when the onset hit me, I had slacked off on my regular exercise and was overeating again, I love warm small bread rolls with dinner, I would eat five or six. I'd have a good meal and then when I got back to my hotel room, I would feel hungry again, so I'd have some chocolate from the bar fridge you know M&M's, Mars Bar, even a Health Bar (really!!!!). It all sounds foolish to me now. I was up for breakfast and had low sugar Weetabix with lite milk and a banana on top, with a cup of tea or coffee. Lunchtime, a Burger or even some Pizza. Sounds good, don't you think? Dinner was anything from the menu, Roast, Fish, Pizza, Meat and usually some salad, as it was healthy and I would always have a side dish of Potato Chips (Fries), I'd finish with two scoops of Ice-cream, again, sounds good don't you think?

I was just another road warrior, and I often see my equivalents in the Novotel's somewhere in the world, with their side dishes of Fries. All of us with a death wish. It's a crazy world out there on the road, and the hotels love us, $7.00 a side dish, from thousands of Road Warriors every evening around the world eating their Fries. Women can be warriors as well……….. Take Joan of Arc as an example.

Here is where the real story commences, suddenly, one night in a hotel overseas I had to get up in the night for a wee (urinate), unusual as this never happened before. I always slept all night with no trouble. The following night it was worse, and by the third night I was up six times. it was crazy. I was heading back home that day, so straight off the flight, and then the 25-kilometre drive home. That afternoon I went to the Doctor, near home, in Northmead Sydney, at that time. We have since moved to the Gold Coast in Queensland.

Here is what transpired in the surgery. Doctor, "Hi Bob, how is it going?" Well, doc it's like this blah blah blah. After he heard the story about me peeing all night, he got up and walked out. Oh, what happened here, where did the Doctor go?

He came back a short time later with a packet in his hand. He opened it, inside was a cute black pouch, he opened the pouch and asked for my finger, pricked my finger with a little plastic tool, took a small tester from the pouch, measured the sample of blood and said "you are a Type 2 Diabetic, your reading is off the map. Best get a blood test, and we will confirm it." "Hence your urination concerns." In my head; Oh, really! It can't be, I've been good with my food of late, no it can't be.

The result should not have been a shock as I had been borderline on Diabetes for years. Probably ten years earlier My wife's uncle, a Chinese Doctor in Korea, told me that was where I was heading many years before. Being a male, I took no notice, and now here I was facing reality, 'holy shit'. (Confusing, a Korean Chinese doctor, however correct he checked me by my pulse, and he was right, amazing. In Chinese medicine pulse taking has been used as one of the most important diagnostic tools for over 2000 years and is considered one of the most valuable of all the methods to which a physician can resort.)

That was not the end of the story. I went back to the Doctor three days later for the results of the blood test. As the peeing had fixed itself, I was hoping like crazy there was not going to be a confirmation of Diabetes. It was probably just a spike, and it would go away. Wrong, the Doctor sat me down and here in the next paragraph is how the one-sided conversation went.

Let's call this "the sentencing". *The Doctor said, "We have received your results, and it confirms that you are a Type 2 Diabetic. Here is your Diabetic's book on what you can eat or suggested meals, it's excellent." The Doctor continued.*

"Well Bob, it's like this you have now been confirmed as a person with Diabetes, so here is what will happen. I have made out a prescription for your new medication, and it will do you for now; however, the dose, will probably increase with time as the diabetes changes and symptoms increase with age. Diabetes will be with you for the remainder of your life, and that life will now probably be shorter. Blood checks, with your free kit, will be necessary every day to monitor how you are going, and you will have to report back to me regularly, once a month. We will do a major blood test every three months. The medication has side effects, and you may feel dizzy or suffer nausea; however, you will adjust. You may be a Type 1 Diabetic before your life is over as your Mother was. You will have to join the National Diabetes Services Scheme (NDSS), as it assists with the cost of your test kit paraphernalia. I'll now be your Doctor for life and will assist you in monitoring the disease, so you stay as well as you can be. By the way, you need to do something about your weight. It's not helping you." (I was thinking, what can I do about my weight, fuck, I have tried everything)

Shit, it was an awful morning, when I came out of the doctors I sat in the car for about 30 minutes in a daze, what happened in there, my life will be shorter and stuffed up by medication and continual blood testing, and it will never stop until I die. Fuck! What a shocking situation. (Excuse my profanities in this book, this is real life, and this is what I said to myself.)

I am a Professional Consultant in the Motor Industry......... that is why I travel so much and spend so much time in hotels. I put a hold on everything that week as I needed time to think about what I could do, if anything. Or should I just sit and get depressed. That almost sounded like a good idea at the time, in fact, the remainder of that day I did exactly that, got depressed!!!!!!

Chapter Seven

WHERE DO I GO FROM HERE?

Warning

Why did I not listen or heed all the signs of Diabetes? If you are reading this book right now, you can start to do something early to prevent this stuff happening to you. You have time, if you are past the point of no return, I am going to tell you what I did to stop all this medical stuff in its tracks, and in doing so, I shocked the local medical people who were advising me to do almost the opposite to what I did do.

Here we go. My personal daily blood sugar testing started the day after the Doctor's official announcement/ confirmation on 27 May 2017. I had to take my blood reading first thing in the morning and 2 hours after every meal. I don't like pricking my fingers or any type of needles, so this was more bad news. I started my medication, and within two hours, I was feeling dizzy and nauseous. If there are side effects, I will get them, and I did. What a bummer, starting my new life, heading for death in an ever so slow manner. Thanks Doc and thanks to Bob (me) for being so stupid and not acting sooner, Prevention is……..and all that stuff. I was very depressed about the self-inflicted situation.

So that first week of my new life as a Type Two Diabetic had started, I was still in shock of some type, numb if you like. About a day or two later, my positive side kicked in, never fails me. I remembered watching a David Letterman interview with Tom Hanks, two people I like. Hanks told Letterman that he had been advised, like me, by his Doctor that he was a Type 2 Diabetic. The conversation went on about how Tom was going to beat this. This conversation had somehow stuck in my head. Unfortunately, Tom never mentioned how he would do it. (Tom was recently on the Gold Coast with his wife at the University Hospital, both were recovering from COVID 19)

The Tom Hanks story sent me to the internet to see what he did. I searched and searched and never found anything. I found reams of other stuff from crazy through to what seemed reasonable. I carried out five days of research and came up with "controlled by diet", as the most practical/understandable information, in the maze of scammers, thieves, crazies and real information, out there. I was eating the recommended meals from my new Diabetes book the Doctor gave me, and it was making little difference to my blood sugar test results, they were worse sometimes. (The Diabetes book would be the perfect paper to start the BBQ with, I discovered later)

Here is the crucial part, after five days of study I settled on a Protein diet. It went against everything that I had learnt in my life and most of what my new diabetes book told me. Hell, Protein diet could kill me as it was all about consuming fat………. could this be correct? My Dad did tell me once about a guy in the UK with a heart condition, he did the reverse of what the doctors recommended, and he survived. During the search, it seemed that the Protein method would be like changing religion, although I have none. From my conclusions, I made up my menu for my meals as I do not have time to cook and imitate the food that I had previously eaten, in what was to be my 'old life'. The web sites are crazy. They are all about making ice-cream that is not ice-cream, pies that are not pies, rice that is not rice. It reminded me of people trying to work out how to make Chicken that tastes like KFC, just go and buy some, silly!!! I was looking for the nuts and bolts of this Protein thing explained for me in simple terms, so now I had my own version. Over a day I broke the food information down, so it was easy for a simple man like me. Now it was time for the human 'Guinea-Pig' to start work.

This segment is very important. Here are the basics. It turns out after days of study that it was simple…….., so simple. That is that Carbohydrates were my new enemy, this I can tell you, as after I stopped sugar in my life Carbohydrates is where I went to satisfy my sugar addiction, and it was subconscious. Again this is so important. I knew that sugar was the killer, yet I never understood that it was the Carbohydrates that were sugars best mate, helping with the sweet crime. Here is a simple example, in the case of a 'Big Mac'. It is the bun that is the real enemy, not the meat, this was **the revolution** for me, yet at this time in my learning, I still did not understand how much difference cutting Carbohydrates would make. It took me over sixty years to find this out, and I have now gifted it to you, *What a guy I am.* (*Send money*) **Conclusion,** sugar is the killer in this murder mystery in its pure form or disguised in a sneaky Carb mask, making you think that it will be a healthy choice for you. I would eat a half a box of Wheat Crackers watching TV in the evening thinking that was good for me, all those lovely healthy seeds in each biscuit. WRONG, Carbs 12.9g in my new world now………. a NO NO.

I still feel stupid missing the Carbohydrates fact for all that time. How cute would I have been in middle life if I had of known this? Very cute, I believe.

Chapter Eight

THE REVOLUTION
(YOU SAY YOU GOT A REAL SOLUTION, BEATLES)

After five days of research, the Human Ginny-Pig was ready, no prep necessary. We had the food, meat, eggs and above ground vegetables precisely what the Low-Carb people were saying. Bacon and eggs for Breakfast, Salad and Ham for lunch, Steak and some green veg for dinner, NICE!!!! I had not consumed bacon for years as it was the enemy in my life, wow it was delicious. So, this was not too bad. After about two weeks of headaches and weakness, my mind started to clear, clearer than I had known for years., and I noticed something. That was………the **craving** after meals for snacks was gone. No real hunger until about four or five hours later, and in the first week, two kilograms had gone? Shit, I could not believe what was happening. I was showing no side effects, just the withdrawal from Carbohydrates in the first two weeks. I had stopped the diabetes medication at the same time I made the change in meals! Your mind does play tricks, as an ex-smoker I know, 2 kilograms disappeared in one week, maybe I now have cancer. Should I stop this crazy diet? No Bob!! Keep going…….. It is the sugar addiction playing tricks on you!

Now, this is where Magic commenced: My blood readings were crashing down at almost a frightening rate. What the hell am I doing to myself? Is this good for me? It was so fast I thought there may be something wrong with me……. maybe I had cancer again, twice now in a matter of days! Can this be correct, I was graphing it in Microsoft Excel and the graph plotting looked like a slippery dip. The charts below show what happened in June, and the Blood Sugar readings were down to normal in 28 days. It was amazing, and they are still normal today. At the same time, my weight loss was moving at warp speed, I was at 115kg, and in three months finished up at 86kg, with my business suits then just hanging off me. I was 88kg this morning it moves up and down by about 2kg.

What I had missed altogether, and I am emphasising this I know, it was the **Carbohydrates** that were causing the weight gain, as the carbohydrates turn to sugar as stated a few paragraphs ago!

I just did not get it. I had replaced the Sugar with Bread Rolls, Wheat Biscuits, Grain Bread, Yogurt Lite, Slim Milk, Bananas, Mangos, Watermelon and all these are Carbohydrate foods. The list goes on and on. I made this my rule 2 in this book. I now look for very low or zero Carbohydrates and Sugar on the food labels, and like me you will be shocked especially with what you read on the lite products information tables. Fruit became much lower on my lists except some berries when I changed to the Low-Carb diet. When I tried those healthy fruit smoothies in 2015, it was a wonder I did not kill myself; my Doctor freaked out when I told him about my new smoothie diet and how much weight I put on. I sold the Nutribullet on eBay the following week.

My Rules

- Rule 1

    My first rule was there would be no exercise in the first three months. It was too hard if I was going to drag around that substantial bodyweight I was carrying. It was better to lose weight first, and then I started the exercise. Now that's a rule you did not expect!

- Rule 2

    I look for very low or zero Carbohydrates and Sugar on the food labels. Carbohydrates replaced with Protein is my success. "I READ THE FOOD LABELS"

- Rule 3

  I was serious about what I was doing, extending my life. I gave up any alcohol. I don't like beer guts, and fortunately, I don't drink much anyway. I include any sugar drink here as a big no no. I minimised the Sugar-Free Coke to about one a week.

- Rule 4

  I must be true/honest to myself if I am going to be successful at this. It was going to be life-changing, that is BIG. I decided to eat to live as the alternative is misery. Simple, some ham, cheese and salad for lunch and you will not be hungry until dinner. (No sugar in the mayo)

- Rule 5

  If I did not measure it, I would not have been able to manage it, so I had a good set of scales and a Blood Sugar test kit (optional). Note: Weight Loss is a daily business!

- Rule 6

  After about three months I restarted my exercise, it is walking in my case. It was easy because I was so much lighter, so I was ready to get out on the road again. Most days I walk about 6 Kilometres along the water. (Exercise is good for blood pressure and just about everything else)

- Rule 7

  I don't just exercise I do what I call "Keep Moving" I clean the garage, fix things on the car, a bit of housework, gardening, even heavy work. Stuff to keep me flexible with movements, as I get older, I must do more than sitting in a chair watching TV. The upshot, "<u>Keep Moving</u>" makes me achieve and feel good.

- Rule 8

  I enjoy life as it is special, and I have made it better and longer.

Here are my first 21 days of Blood Sugar Readings, amazing I reckon!

BS First 21 Days				
Date	Wake-Up	After Breakfast	2Hrs After Lunch	2Hrs After dinner
Saturday, 27 May 2017	11.0	18.0	14.7	9.3
Sunday, 28 May 2017	11.6	12.8	14.2	10.3
Monday, 29 May 2017	12.7	9.5	12.6	13.5
Tuesday, 30 May 2017	10.8	8.9	11.3	8.3
Wednesday, 31 May 2017	9.3	10.0	7.4	8.6
Thursday, 1 June 2017	9.5	8.6	7.9	7.9
Friday, 2 June 2017	7.9	7.8	8.4	7.7
Saturday, 3 June 2017	6.9	7.4	6.3	6.7
Sunday, 4 June 2017	7.7	7.4	6.9	6.3

Monday, 5 June 2017	6.2	7.6	7.0	8.8
Tuesday, 6 June 2017	7.3	7.6	7.8	8.5
Wednesday, 7 June 2017	7.2	7.1	6.6	6.9
Thursday, 8 June 2017	7.5	8.6	6.8	6.7
Friday, 9 June 2017	6.6	7.0	6.4	6.4
Saturday, 10 June 2017	6.8	7.7	7.0	7.0
Sunday, 11 June 2017	6.0	6.6	6.0	6.5
Monday, 12 June 2017	5.7	6.0	5.9	7.0
Tuesday, 13 June 2017	5.5	7.0	5.8	6.1
Wednesday, 14 June 2017	5.8	6.0	5.8	6.4
Thursday, 15 June 2017	5.8	6.4	6.4	6.7
Friday, 16 June 2017	6.0	6.4	5.7	6.2
7 More Days and Normal				
Saturday, 17 June 2017	5.8	6.1	5.9	5.3
Sunday, 18 June 2017	5.3	6.3	5.4	5.5
Monday, 19 June 2017	5.1	5.5	5.8	4.8
Tuesday, 20 June 2017	5.2	5.4	5.5	4.8
Wednesday, 21 June 2017	5.1	5.5	5.3	7.0
Thursday, 22 June 2017	5.0	4.9	5.1	5.9
Friday, 23 June 2017	5.0	5.5	5.5	5.2

I had been in this position previously when I stopped sugar, with the weight loss coming off in a hurry. The question was, could I maintain/sustain the weight loss and the reduction in Blood Sugar, if I could not, I would not be able to write this book. It is exactly three years as I write this and I'm still not a Type 2 Diabetic, the overall readings came back up a little over the two years, and then settled down to normal, I was 5.8 this morning for example. And I was 87.0Kg's this morning when I weighed myself.

People kept telling me that as you get older, you can't lose weight as the young ones can. Yes, well, that is BS, and I have proved it. It is not age-related, it is determination related, with a genuine want to live longer.

Two things like good friends, travel together………… weight and blood sugar If I go off track, I can see the immediate kilogram gain, usually one or two (kg) so I then just pull back, so I understand where the sugar is coming from, which food, that is. Blood Sugar testing, 2 hours after meals, tells me this quickly, that is, which foods are causing concerns.

So, my research method is unusual, as I use the blood sugar readings to identify who's labels on carbohydrates are incorrect or inconsistent. I'm not recommending this method; however, for me, it makes it all the more accurate. For those who do not have Diabetes, they may choose to follow the protein method only.

What has to happen is, the old saying you have to eat to live, so, it may be boring, yet I am going to be healthier and live longer even though the stuff I will be eating, is what they tell you not to eat. I cleaned my section of the pantry out of things with Lite, High Carb and Sugar on the labels.

Finally! (Proof)

Finally, in this section, my first blood test after three months in my new world of weight loss and low Blood Sugar came in and proved I was not diabetic anymore and it was the most normal blood test I could remember. My latest blood tests show a very slight rise in Cholesterol; however, nothing to worry about, the remainder is normal. Some instant things that happened at the three months goalpost were, less body swelling, less acid stomach, blood pressure excellent, more energy and no side effects except constipation from time to time (Psyllium Husk Caps fixed that). Hey, let's call this a win win! My Doctor said I could stop the medication. I told him I stopped on day two, three months prior. Interesting look on the doctors' face during that visit.

Chapter Nine

A DAY IN THE LIFE
(BEATLES)

So, what is life like in this new world? How do I travel and eat? What about a day out in the boat? What do I eat overall? What do others say and think about the changes I have made?

Well, life is not too bad or too hard as the first thing is my disposition has always been positive. Those genes are an excellent place to start. When I do go down (depression) it is usually only for a day then I get up fighting. **This sentence is BIG, the thing about a protein diet is that you are not hungry in between meals, so it takes away that stress of wanting something to eat all the time. This is the base secret of Low-Carb.** I like living, I have never needed things to get me high, waking in the morning in my beautiful Australia is a gift that so many in the world would wish for, and I have it.

I can do what I like now, as my diet is simple, moreover I can find Protein anywhere......... it's easy. I did not think finding the right food when I was out and about would be that simple. I have found that the worst thing that can happen is eating a nude burger, no buns just the content.

Travel, and I have to do this often, is not a barrier. Writing this, travel currently is off due to COVID 19; however, I'll give you a typical example below.

Away to Brisbane Airport at 4:30 am
Check-in and through Customs at 5:45 am
Good breakfast in the club at 6 am Bacon, Tomato & Egg
3-hour flight to Auckland arrive at about 2 pm Big Mac and black coffee at the airport. Just eat the centre and bin the bun.
To the hotel
Dinner at 7 pm Lamb-Shank and steamed vegetable. Yum

As you can see, it is very easy, and I'm not hungry after the meals so no raiding the mini bar in the hotel room. I can't tell you exactly what to eat, you can work that out, just Low-Carb and Protein, more rough examples of my diet following.

What about at home:

Breakfast: Bacon, Tomato & Fried Eggs, Coffee with thick cream. (Just two teaspoons of cream).
Lunch: Ham, cheese and salad, no bread, and black coffee.
Dinner: Low Carb Pork Sausages, cheese and salad or vegetables and black tea.

What about a day out in the boat?

Breakfast: Bacon, Tomato & Fried Eggs, Coffee black. (at the marina restaurant).
Lunch: Nude (no Bun) Burger at the Burger shop at Paradise Point, delicious. Coffee with thick cream onboard the boat. (Just two teaspoons of cream).
Dinner: Fillet Steak, BBQ vegetables. Yum. And black coffee.

That's it…… easy, don't you think? You are smart, so protein food suggestions are listed all over the internet, so it's straightforward for you to find. I have included some simple charts in the back of this publication.

So, what do others think, to be honest, I don't care; however, it was strange at first. About four people who know me well were very concerned and took me aside, in each case, they asked me if I had cancer. So, if you travel this path, you will have some questions asked. The detractors told me it would not work, and it is dangerous............ I am still here! As I said, I am not concerned what they think, that is not the reason I am doing it, its very simple......... I just want to live longer.

I know I keep saying it, here I go again. It's all about sugar and low carbs. How do I know if my diet is working correctly? Easy, I am not hungry between meals. If I become hungry between meals, there may be sugar sneaking into my diet somewhere, so I go over what I'm doing with food and don't lie to myself. As can be seen in this book I am a sugar addict, and its not easy withdrawing. To confirm what I am eating is not doing me harm, I measure my blood sugar two hours after meals. I soon know what is going on.

Here are some personal experiences.

Fat

My days of worrying about the danger of fat are over, as I need fat in my diet every day as that is where my energy comes from. The fat replaces the sugar. Hence the bacon every morning cooked in butter. My Cholesterol has not altered much, it was never high, and I now believe that sugar is going to kill me before the fat will. I know, where is the proof? You can make your own decisions on Low-

Carb & Fat after your own research. Here is something to think about regarding proof, I was overweight, very high blood pressure, snoring, out of breath, acid stomach, willpower exhausted, feeling like a looser and now a Type 2 Diabetic, I am not anymore! My blood tests are excellent, and I am still not a diabetic after three years on Low Carb. From two random guys/gals, one thin and on a protein diet, the other is large/overweight and on an eating anything diet, who will live the longest? There are not many fat guys in old people's homes. I rest my case again, as I did earlier in the book's introduction.

Antibiotics

When I got the flu and an infected throat, the Doctor said it was a good idea if I take a one-week course of antibiotics. About halfway through the week, my blood sugar was gradually going up, higher and higher. When it got to 7.8, I had to do something, and my diet was excellent, so the only difference was the tablets. I was now well enough, so I put the brakes on and stopped the pills. Gradually the blood sugar came down again to normal. So, this may not apply to everyone; however, it sure affected me, so be careful.

Peanuts Salted

Be careful of peanuts they are moreish. Pistachio's and Cashews are on the bad end of the scale. Other nuts refer to the simple chart at the back of the book.

Cream

I had cream in my coffee, and my Blood Sugar would spike sometimes, cream should be pure fat, however, to me it appears that cream is different batch to batch and brand to brand, so I reduced the coffee with cream to two cups a day with cream. I found my blood sugar results were the most consistent with the more expensive brands. The human Guineapig solved the issue again.

Vegetables

As you will learn, the lowest carb vegetables are above ground. However, I do have a small amount of carrot with salad. Where I am very careful is with Restaurants and Hotel meals. Every so often vegetables give me a blood sugar spike, as I think they put sugar in the water they cook the vegetables in, which makes them taste better, I guess.

Sugar/Carb Free Coke

No Sugar Coke does not affect my blood sugar. I don't drink much, as I don't know what else is in it?

Chewing Gum

Chewing sugar-free gum has a small effect on Blood Sugar if I chew too much. I don't know why. I like gum, so I have a tiny amount once every few days and make it last for a long time.

Sugar-free mints are okay in my case. However, I must watch myself as they make me feel like I want more sugar.

Pork Sausages

Pork Sausages, Coles in Australia. I have them about twice a week. I do a BBQ 1 or 2, and they don't spike my blood sugar at all.

Milk

Milk is so so. I sometimes put one of those small long-life hotel or airline containers in my coffee to make it taste better. No spikes so far!!

Tea and coffee black

Tea and coffee black have zero effect on my blood sugar.

Lite/Light

This one is easy I eat or drink nothing lite as it is a hoax. That hoax helped me get to where I did with Type Two Diabetes. Thanks a lot! I check the carbs on everything I pick up. I tend not to eat anything above 3g Carbs. I don't trust if I start putting weight back on it will be from something that has sugar in it. I track my food so I can identify the culprit, like the antibiotics, it was easy to spot.

Worst Places

The worst place of all for me is the supermarket. Why? As I can see 60 years of my old life spread out before me, high sugar, high carb everywhere, Weatbix with a Banana was heaven, fruit delicious mango's, cake, candy, chocolate. I get in and out of the supermarket as quickly as I can.

Another problem area is Coffee Shops Those displays with the Carrot Cake, Lemon Meringue Pie, and you know the rest. I get in and out as quickly as I can.

Hotels Restaurants with all that food on the menu, when I am travelling, many times I go out and buy some stuff at the supermarket, for example, Smoked Salmon and salad. Or I have a meal sent to the room. I was a lover of bread rolls, so I keep away from them, everyone has them sitting on their sides plates when you are in the main hotel eating areas. It's horrible.

Chapter Ten

WHEN YOU HIT THE WALL

When you hit the wall, as I did on that day in May 2017, I had only one question to ask myself. The question was: Who is the only person that matters here right now? This sound very self-centred, and it was. I'm still here now because of that decision to focus for that one week. That's all ....one week.

Before you go on - what thoughts does this self-centeredness conjure up for you? Stop! I will leave you to work it out.

I believe that our bodies are much like an ecosystem. As such, if any part of our body is 'out of wack' the entire ecosystem suffers. Often this shows up as sickness and in the worst cases killing us, and as they say, probably STRESS, (being our mental health), is important as one the worst body ecosystem destroyers........... we know. As we put on more body weight, this adds to our silent stress, this eats away at us mentally, exacerbating where we are heading. Then we eat more of our favourite sugar food to help forget what we are doing to ourselves. It's a crazy cycle that keeps spinning us around with the centrifugal force sending us to the black dog. (Depression)

Many will recognise this situation.

Sometimes this ecosystem event comes about from a singular shocking event. An example would be recovering from COVID-19, it will take many years to repair the damage done to the body ecosystem, for millions of people around the world.

In my case, the root cause, carbs/sugar was hard to pin down, though the symptoms came out everywhere.

Around the world, there are many examples of ecosystems being gradually destroyed for example in Australia Dingo's being killed off when they are a vital link. Bringing them back in some areas restored the system in the main. In America's Yellowstone Park, the Grey Wolves were returned to correct the eco-balance. The thing here is it's like our body's, and we can make changes that restore the ecosystem, it is just a matter of learning what to do.

My job it turned out to be was to restore my balance, in my ecosystem, that is made up of many components; Food, Exercise, Environment, Stress, Love, Work, and

Relaxation as examples. I am not perfect; however, I have made tremendous progress.

I was stuck at this point, and I was failing to address my body's needs and indirectly letting down my complete ecosystem. It's like this; the rivers run dry or flood; there is erosion, some areas start to die. A weak ecosystem makes it easier for predators to get into the system bringing infection virus's, etc., and they are difficult to fight if the body is run-down.

We can survive and perhaps even thrive, yet it seems for many of us, we eventually stall, if we don't focus on health. So, my wish is, that my readers don't leave the awareness until it's too late, thus allowing the sugar to do its dirty work.

I know, this seems like a bit of a crazy notion. What if you got some simplicity around this idea and applied it to your health?

- What would that mean?
- What would that change?
- How would you think differently about your health?
- How would you transform your health, approach?
- What would you measure to understand, progress?

See, by simply asking the question, you will pursue an answer.

This book is about how to gain balance. It is a short selfish diversion that corrected my entire ecosystem with amazing results. The hard work part for me was only about two weeks at the start, yet it was worth it for me, and those around me.

Chapter Eleven

DOCTORS

In my case, this became tricky, and my Doctor did not understand what was happening. He had never seen anything like it, and astonishment was the response I observed. His surprise was only equalled by my own. In the finish, he was very impressed.

I moved from the state of New South Wales to Queensland so could not take my Doctor with me. Thus, began the search for a new Doctor.

When it comes to Low-Carb, there were not many doctors who were willing to listen or understand what I had achieved. I tried many, and only after almost three years found a GP who specialises in Low-Carb.

Here are some of the things that happened to me:

I have a heart Check every two years, the Heart Specialist got very angry with me and told me my diet was not that good, and anyone could reverse Diabetes with all types of foods. It was no use debating with this guy he was locked in. Other GP's I saw were not interested; however; they had found a new thing to blame for my general ailments, Low-Carb. In the finish, I stopped telling them I was on a Low-Carb diet as it just caused unnecessary debate, and they liked to win. That is okay I'll let them think what they like.

I finally found a Low-Carb Doctor within walking distance of my home, that fixed it. All it took was a search on Google, then a bit of research on what people were saying about the individual GP's and that solved my situation.

My belief now is, it is no use trying to convince the medical people about Low-Carb, it is better too, "let it be", as Paul Mcarthy's Mother said, then move to a doctor who understands. This debate will be around for years as it is an enormous change for the professionals. They are so entrenched that only their methods can solve weight loss, and most believe there is no way to reverse Diabetes.

Chapter Twelve

THE LARGE CHOPSTICKS AND SCISSORS
(APPROACHING CHANGE)

I would like to start this chapter with some logic and how we are not willing to see things from another point of view and how difficult it is to change that view. Set in our ways if you like of not accepting change or a better way. With change there are two sides, a plus and minus if you like. You must be willing to give something away to gain something new. So, it is a transaction you make to improve one's life.

This is about my first time in Asia, which was a business trip to Seoul and Ulsan Korea. I had been to the UK and the US before, however nowhere in the Asian region. My brother had primed me telling me Korea was a third world experience so you can imagine what I was thinking prior to the trip.

As we came in over Seoul from Tokyo, I was expecting

an airport that looked like Alice Springs in 1979. However, after landing at Kimpo Airport, to my surprise, there were other planes lined up and there was more air traffic, buildings and people than in Tokyo where I had just arrived from. When we cleared customs and got outside there were so many cars and the traffic as we drove into central Seoul was like nothing I had ever seen before. It is a huge city. Freeways crisscrossing the city, skyscrapers, crowds, shops everywhere, street cafés, tent dine in meals and markets. Third world, I don't think so!!!!!

I was very much like a child as I traveled with Korean people for the first time; as I knew nothing about the culture. On the second day we were taken to lunch at a restaurant not far from the Olympic Stadium in Seoul (the Olympics had just finished). The restaurant was a Korean Barbeque House, which are very popular in Korea. I was with a Korean guy called Mr. Kim and some other business colleagues (Mr. Kim will know who I am talking about, as he is now a lifelong dear friend). For those who don't know, the surname Kim is a far more common name in Korea than Smith is in Australia, America, or UK.

The restaurant was a pleasant place with a genuine Asian feel which I came to love over the years. You had to take your shoes off at the door and of course from that moment the service was superb (we can learn something just from this). At that time, I could not use chopsticks at all, so I had my own problems that lunch time. I also had to sit on the floor with my legs crossed which was painful after a very short time. I now know to look for Korean restaurants with a pit or hole under the table where you can put your legs.

A strange thing occurred in the restaurant. The waitress brought out sliced steak on a large metal tray and with very large chopsticks. Who could be the person who was going to use these? I had never seen chopsticks that big in my life (as a matter of fact, I had not seen many chopsticks at all except those in the local Chinese takeaway). Also, on the plate was a pair of scissors. What would these be for? Was someone going to do some sewing or cutting paper?!

After we settled in, Mr. Kim started with his advice to me. It was a little serious as I did not know him and I was trying to do all the right things to please my newfound Asian friends. I was so worried about the culture and insulting someone as I had heard so many stories: 'don't blow your nose near these people'; 'don't write on their business cards';' don't stab any fool with a chopstick' and so on. Mr Kim asked in a serious tone if I could use chopsticks, so I told him I could not. He asked would I like to try. I was polite, so I asked if he could arrange a fork. He told me he could not and would not assist me with a fork.

In my mind I said, shit, and asked myself who is this guy and what is going on here. This was a serious situation; my first meal in Asia and I was in for an argument with the host. I did not realise, but it was going to get more serious.

Mr. Kim proceeded to tell me if I could not use chopsticks then I would go hungry. Yes, it was getting more serious. Mr. Kim then made me an offer. He would teach me how to use them, right there and then, that way I would not starve. Shit is he serious?! Here I am in Korea for my first lunch with a worldwide senior executive and I am about to stuff it up completely.

Then I got it. This guy had a sense of humor and a good one. He played me well and still does to this day. Many times, over the years we have laughed together about this first meeting and have had many other comical times together. (Remember that when you deal in Asia or with Asian people, they love fun and humor as well). Yes, he taught me that day to use not just chopsticks, he taught me how to use thin chrome chopsticks and I have never looked back. I probably have been using them more than western utensils ever since. I accepted change and made a good friend in the process.

Once we had all settled down for the meal a girl came out to cook it. Yes, she used the large chopsticks so that she was far enough away from the heat to not burn herself. Once the steak on the BBQ was almost done, she used the scissors to cut it up. I have to say that I had a problem accepting this as my Mum used scissors for sewing and somehow, I just could not see why they should be used for cutting meat. Something was wrong with this. I tried to find a reason why they should not be used. It was not hygienic (a knife is more practical) and they are not designed for this purpose.

Now I think about it realistically. How smart was it? It is so easy to cut up meat with scissors. It is so practical and yet I had trouble accepting it as my mother never did it and used scissors for sewing and cutting wrapping paper yet not in food preparation.

That was a good day. I learnt to use chopsticks (thin chrome chopsticks) and that scissors are an excellent tool for cutting food. Both these things I use today (thank you Mr. Kim). So, accepting change can be good, as it was in this case. What would have happened if I blocked myself to this change? I would have not learnt. And when you stop learning and stop trying new things you gradually spiral towards killing your mind. The mind needs this exercise just like your body needs exercise.

To arrive at this Low-Carb diet, I had to be opened minded and be willing to change. The story in this chapter was to show how we can block our minds. I did, as you can see and, three things changed, all nationalities have humor so we can share it, Large Chop Sticks are not stupid they are very practical, we have them is our kitchen and Scissors are an excellent tool when cooking.

With my Low Carb Diet, I was on the edge and at first ,doubted it, however, I took the risk, learnt and I am still here. This change saw me give up many foods I loved in exchange for a longer healthier life, I accepted these changes and it made me much happier and healthier.

Put off for one day and ten days will pass.

- *Korean Proverb*

Chapter Thirteen

IF I WERE YOU

I can't tell anyone what to do, all I can tell you is what I did and the success, and if you can learn from this, it is good. Will it work for you, I don't know, yet I cannot see why it should not work if you follow the Protein way, wherever the information is sourced. The main thing is that you have found someone who has done it, and more importantly, it has sustained with only positive side effects.

Why would you not want to stay alive, I go down to the Broadwater here on the Gold Coast every day. It fills my heart & soul. I was confined for 14 days after coming back from overseas. I sat out the back every day with a coffee first thing and watched the local birds. The birds get up every day, and they are positive and happy, singing, talking, playing, and just before they go to bed, there is a massive conversation about what happened in the day. Plus, they eat to live apart from the occasional greedy Seagull or Pigeon. They have got it right!!!!~!

I do not have to; however, as most days, I do my Blood Sugar, especially if I've been eating out. In business, we call this a KPI, so the blood test is my Key Performance Indicator, and it has been since my discovery that I was a Type Two Diabetic back in 2017.

Chapter Fourteen:

IN THE BEGINNING
MY PLAN

Here is the plan I used to begin reversing the Diabetes, back then, I had little faith it would work; however, as you read, it worked and fast. Part of my plan was a Protein meal plan for a week. This was so I could repeat it, Week in Week out. The second table below is the meals. It is almost the same today.

My Simple 10 Step Plan (When all this unravelled)	
1	I researched everything I could find on the internet over a one-week period, I had then identified the best options, so I was ready to go. A big risk however but I pushed ahead.
2	I selected a start date; it was easy. I decided on the following Monday after my internet research.
3	I made sure the first two weeks were clear of high workload. I knew I was going to suffer withdrawal. Some of the side effects were weakness, a bit dizzy and lethargic as I understood at that time. (It was true)
4	I Purchased a good set of scales, and in my case, a good quality Blood Sugar Test Kit, the one the Doctor supplied free was rubbish. (If it can't measure it you can't manage it.)

5	I set up a way to records my Weight, Blood Sugar, Blood Pressure, Food daily, using a Word spreadsheet (It could have been an exercise book.) I included a graph on Blood Sugar and Weight.
6	Blood Sugar, I planned (as the Doctor advised me to) first thing in the morning and 2 hours after meals.
7	Weight, I planned to measure every day after my shower in the mornings and Blood Pressure the same, for consistency. (Blood pressure was for my interest only, to ensure it was not going up with the significant change I was making)
8	I recorded progress for three months up to the Blood Test that was to confirm I was still a diabetic, it confirmed I was not. (I fooled them)
9	I focused on being honest with myself, or this would not work, I could not cheat as the measurement would catch me.
10	I continued what I was doing for a further three months to prove it worked and it did. I then continued to this day.

As can be seen, it was simple, I still measure my weight every morning and my Blood Sugar, it is not necessary to record it anymore as I can see what food is impacting on my diet.

Below is an idea of my diet even today, my wife made me a lovely omelette tonight with beautiful Korean mushrooms and a small amount of cheese yum, yum.

My Simple 7 Day Food Plan (When all this unravelled) Plus Measurement

Weight KG	88	87	86.5
Exercise	5.2km	6.0km	4.5km Gardening
Drinks/ Snacks	Few nuts Black Coffee at the Qantas Club	2 Black Coffee	2 Black Coffee & Cream
BS After Dinner	4.6	5.2	5.3
Dinner	Silverside with Salad	Streak and vegetables	Streak and Steamed vegetables
BS After Lunch	5.3	5.4	5.3
Lunch	Tuna Salad Black Coffee	KFC skin removed	KFC skin removed, Coke No Sugar
BS After Breakfast	6.3	5.8	6.0
Breakfast	Bacon-Eggs & Black Coffee	Fried Eggs, Fried tomato & Fried Bacon with Coffee	Fried Eggs, Fried tomato & Fried Bacon with Coffee/Cream
BS	6.7	5.1	5.3

87	88	89	88.5
6.0km	6.0km	5.0km	6.0km
Very small dish of Salted peanus — 5.2	Tiny dish of Salted peanuts & Coffee — 5.5	2 Black Coffee & Cream — 5.6	2 Black Coffee — 5.7
BBQ Steak & Salad with Coffee/Cream — 5.4	Ham, Tomato and Cheese Omelette with Salad — 5.3	BBQ Lamb & Salad with Coffee/Cream — 5.5	BBQ Fish & Salad with Coffee — 5.6
Ham Salad with Coffee — 5.4	Tuna Salad with Coffee — 5.7	Big Mac no Buns with salad and Black Coffee — 5.6	Ham Salad with Coffee — 5.5
Scrabbles Eggs, Fried tomato & Fried Bacon with Coffee — 5.8	Fried Eggs, Fried tomato & Fried Bacon with Coffee/Cream — 5.9	Scrabbles Eggs, Fried tomato & Fried Bacon with Coffee — 5.8	Fried Eggs, Fried tomato & Fried Bacon with Coffee — 6.0

Chapter Fifteen

THE FINAL WORD

My eating disorder, (as I call it sometimes), was caused by a combination of factors......... the factors being an English background and the fact that when I was younger.......... we saw no danger in sugar as it was normal. (Like Smoking) This food saw me travel through life well until the midlife stress of family plus work hit. This part of my life, I realised that I had to exercise and watch my blood pressure and I never related anything to food, yet I was putting on weight. Looking back, I was one of those people who could eat anything and have no weight gain. This advantage disappeared.

The total combination was, giving up smoking, travelling for work, love of sugar and laziness. I finished up with the sugar addiction being as strong as smoking and more persuasive, that is, my mind got to the tricky/ sneaky stage looking for sugar in anything thus I was seeking out the carbohydrate, and I did not know. Lite and low sugar, grain, fruit, it all sounded so right and so healthy, yet it was killing me.

Let's finish with a sobering end, in 2007. I was going through Perth Airport and almost collapsed on the floor as I dragged my bag across the carpet section of the airport to the check-in. I was puffing and feeling terrible. In the QANTAS Club, I sat and pondered what happened and thought this was the onset of old age. Back in Sydney, they found I had a heart concern. In the hospital, they found one blocked artery and fitted a stent, quick and easy and back to normal. (My Dad would have lived to 100 if this was available when he was alive)

Now here is the final thing for you the reader to ponder, in my life, I have never had a cholesterol concern, yet, they told me Cholesterol was the cause of the blocked artery. The Specialist and my GP had no explanation. I do have the answer, and it is the only conclusion that I can come to, sugar, my addiction caused it. Its sugar that gummed up my artery's.

Due to business, I am regularly in a social setting where food and drink are plentiful. People ask why I don't drink:

One: it is because I was drunk twice on Beer when I was in my late teens and never again did I want that horrible feeling of spinning then vomiting. (Port and

Whisky after that)

Two: I saw so many drinking businesspeople ruin their careers by making fools of themselves, plus they would blow away company money and make foolish decisions.

Thee: I saw a drunk young man fall 10 metres off a balcony and suffer a severe brain injury, his life finished even though he lived, the happiness he felt that night due to the drink turned to an empty life, so unfortunate.

Four: Very basic, I love life; I love the mornings and drink can steal that away from me.

Note: My wife and I have a Port wine on exceptional occasions. I don't hate drink just respect what it can do to my health and safety.

Here are the two words I used every day to arrive at Weight and Blood Sugar sustainability: Determination and Persistence. In this situation there is one clear decision that I made, unlike *the Terminator or General MacArthur (I'll Be Back/I Shall Return)* there was/is no going back as even a binge surge of sugar can be risky.

I'm signing off, living in Australia near the water on the Gold Coast is a gift that I appreciate every day.

Walking along the Broadwater is my Drink, Drugs, Love, Meditation, Visually Pleasing and giving a Feeling of Freedom, The people the birds, the dogs, the fish and the Dolphins down there every day agree with me, I believe.

Appendix

Some Simple Charts below that may assist.

Drinks	Good	Not so Good	Poor	Comments
Water	√			
Water with lemon	√			
Coffee	√			No Sugar or Milk, With Cream is okay however, some cream has sugar in it.
Tea	√			No Sugar or Milk
Diet soft drink	√			Makes you feel like having more sugar
Wine		√		Half glass is enough
Coconut water		√		Never tried this
Vegetable juice		√		Above ground Vegetables
Milk			√	Especially long life you can taste the sugar in the cheap brands
Soy milk			√	
Beer			√	
Coffee made with milk e.g.Cappuccino			√	
Orange juice			√	

			√	
Energy drink			√	
Ice tea			√	
Soft drink			√	
Smoothie			√	I had crazy weight gain with this years ago.
Milkshake			√	No, No, No; because I love a banana one with malt

Vegetables Carbs				
Type	**Good**	**Not so Good**	**Poor**	**Comments**
Asparagus	√			
Avocado	√			
Beetroot		√		
Broccoli	√			
Brussels sprouts		√		
Cabbage	√			
Capsicum (Peppers)		√		The yellow colour is higher Carb
Carrot	√			
Cauliflower	√			
Cucumber	√			
Eggplant	√			
Green beans	√			
Kale	√			

Lettuce	√			
Olives	√			
Onion		√		
Parsnip		√		
Potato			√	
Spinach	√			
Sweet potato			√	
Zucchini	√			

Fruit

Type	Good	Not so Good	Poor	Comments
Banana			√	
Blackberry	√			
Blueberry			√	
Cherries			√	
Coconut			√	
Grapes			√	
Kiwi fruit			√	
Lemon		√		
Mandarin			√	
Mango			√	
Orange			√	
Pawpaw		√		

	Good	Not so Good	Poor	
Peach			√	
Pears			√	
Pineapple			√	
Plum		√		
Raspberry	√			
Strawberry	√			
Watermelon		√		

Nuts

Type	Good	Not so Good	Poor	Comments
Peanuts		√		
Brazil	√			
Cashew			√	
Hazel		√		
Macadamia	√			
Pecan	√			
Pine nuts		√		
Pistachio			√	
Wallnut	√			

Snack & Some Breakfast Food

Type	Good	Not so Good	Poor	Comments
Avocado	√			

Cheese	√		
Cold sliced meat	√		
Corn Chips		√	
Cornflakes		√	
Eggs	√		
Olives	√		
Potato Chips		√	
Wheat Biscuits		√	
Cereal Overall		√	

BOB MOSS

https://weight-loss.management
info@weight-loss.management

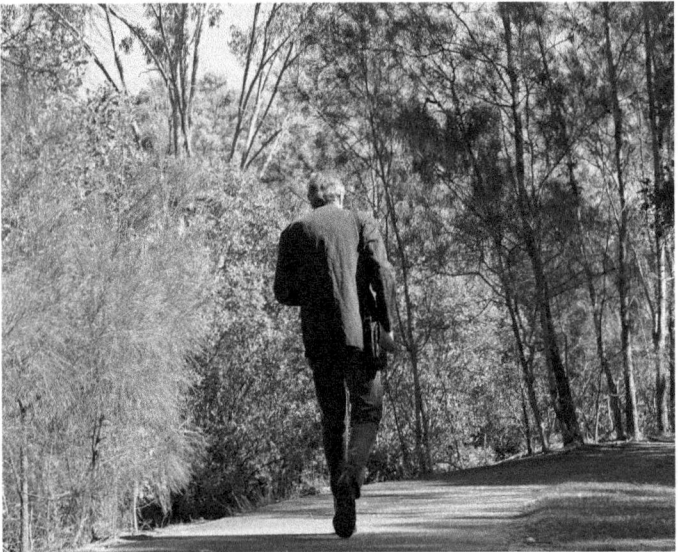